HEALTHY RECIPES TO LOOSE WEIGHT

Top fat burning foods with weight loss tips

The best 32 vegetable recipes

Katharina Morell

I0426363

Published by:

JoelNoah S.A.

info@joelnoah.com

Author: Katharina Morell

HEALTHY RECIPES TO LOOSE WEIGHT

Top fat burning foods with weight loss tips

The best 32 vegetable recipes

ISBN-13: 978-1494222116

ISBN-10: 1494222116

Copyright 2013 by JoelNoah S.A.

CONTENTS

Introduction

During the last 20 years, diseases such as diabetes type II, heart attacks, strokes, Alzheimer, problems with the joints, cancer and metabolic disorders increased explosively.

A healthy nutrition is the key to well-being, an ideal weight, and a life in which diseases have virtually no role.

Many of our meals consist of inferior preprocessed foods or "bad" carbohydrates, which greatly increase the blood sugar level and ultimately cause overweight and the diseases named above.

The foods and recipes described in this book will let you lose your excess fat naturally way, without going hungry, and will thus let you live a very healthy life.

The recipes and recipe suggestions listed will ensure that there will be no boredom on your daily menu. Be creative, and try to prepare a meal from the recipes suggested.

Even if you don't have the time or the desire to cook, in this book you'll find sufficient suggestions to have delicious meals quickly on your table.

Why are so many people overweight?

Almost 60% of the population living in Europe and the States are overweight. Not just because they eat too much, but also because they eat the wrong food. Apart from disrupted eating habits, metabolic disorders, a lack of exercise and genetic factors, an incorrect nutrition has by far the greatest influence on overweight.

Nowadays only 20% of our food comes from nature; the remaining 80% are from industry, are preprocessed foods, artificial aromas or other chemically manufactured products.

Please take a look at all the packaged foods in your kitchen. At the end of the list of ingredients, you'll find names that sound like chemicals, or codes that start with "E". These are artificial additives, preservatives, binders, flavor enhancers and pigments. Our body was not made to use these substances effectively, and that's exactly what robs it of its energy and impetus, and results in a disrupted metabolism. These additives are stored in fat cells together with all the extra calories ingested.

Preprocessed foods, labeled as "no cholesterol", "light", or other descriptions, are shams. It is precisely these products that make the body "sick", and the person fat.

Make me – and yourself – an important favor. Look carefully in your kitchen for all of these products, and get rid of them.

That way, you'll have done the first great step to lose weight successfully.

The objective is to provide our body with 100% of the required vitamins, minerals, and macronutrients, to bring the body back into balance and to bring the metabolism up to full speed.

You'll get a healthy weight for your size and body build, and a well-working digestion, intake and excretion. All of these factors will result in you having an excellent weight and no more trouble with weight loss, and your general constitution will become noticeably better.

Foods you should avoid

The human body is a product of evolution, that is, it has developed for thousands of years. This is the reason that you should only consume natural foods which the human body has recognized as useful for thousands of years.

For example, did you know that margarine and similar low-fat spreads are so similar, in their structure, to plastics, that they remain "fresh" longer than butter or oils?

Avoid artificial fats such as margarine, grease sprays, low-fat spreads, etc.

Or did you realize that our body only recognizes the product sugar as such for ca. 250 years? Previously, people used mainly honey as a sweetener, if they used sweeteners at all. Nowadays, we find sugar in practically any processed product (ketchup, mustard, muesli, cocoa, cookies, syrup, lemonade, etc.).

Among other things, sugar is also used as a preservative.

In small quantities (a few grams per day), sugar can even be healthy, and helps against constipation, flatulence and colic. However, on average we consume over 100 grams of sugar a day; that's much more than what is actually healthy. This puts a great strain on our pancreas, and the blood insulin level, responsible for hunger attacks, is extremely high. A high insulin level in the blood prevents the body from burning excess fat.

Please remember: if you consume sugar, the body will not burn fat, and you won't lose weight.

Try to avoid sugar (glucose, glucose syrup, sucrose); there is a great alternative for sugar, namely stevia.

Stevia is a natural sweetener. It is 300 times as sweet as sugar, and appropriate for diabetics. The stevia that you can purchase in natural food stores or bio-stores is usually available in a weakened form. Stevia is a plant from South America, used by Paraguayan and Peruvian Indians for hundreds of years as a sweetener and its assumed medical properties. You can also buy stevia over the Internet. Just type "stevia" into Google, and you'll see a list of shops that offer it.

Stevia is available in different forms, as powder, drops, tablets and extract. In the USA it was already officially allowed, and many manufacturers (Pepsi, among others) are gradually changing their products to use stevia.

Simply use stevia according to your taste (but remember that just one drop is enormously sweet). Just put one to two drops into your tea, when you would normally use a teaspoon of sugar. When baking, adapt the amount to the recipes. If you experiment a bit with stevia, you'll quickly find out how much you need to use to replace the sugar you used previously.

Also try to remove artificial sugar such as aspartame (trademarks include Nutrasweet and Canderel) from your list. You will find aspartame in diet products such as diet lemonade, sugar-free chewing gum, sugar-free peppermint bonbons, etc. I will go a step further and claim that aspartame promotes the formation of cancer!

You should likewise avoid white flour products such as bread, buns, cookies, cakes, pastas, etc.

With these products, the starch molecules bring the insulin level to a maximum. We now know that a high insulin level in your blood is bad for your health and hinders the process of losing weight.

Better consume whole grain bread or whole grain products; your body will be grateful for this.

Please remember: When you consume white flour products, your body won't burn fat, and you won't lose weight.

If up until now you ate white flour bread with butter and a piece of cheese or sausage, you should know that:

The insulin level in the blood goes up.

Butter, cheese and sausage will be stored directly in your hips as fat.

Did you know that in the list of valuable foods, the wheat flour that has been grinded out is way down? It has but little nutritional value, and is an insidious fattener. You'll find this fattener in the following products: toast, cookies, hamburger bread, gourmet baguettes, pretzel sticks, instant soup, frozen pizza, breadsticks, warmed up rolls, etc.

Additional fatteners include refined "white" carbohydrates such as white rice (long corn rice, milk rice, etc.) and traditional noodles from durum wheat semolina.

Refrain from eating French fries, fried potatoes, instant puree, frozen gratin, instant meatballs, potato pancakes, casserole and chips. The combination of fat and carbohydrates works as a calorie bomb for your body.

You might be asking yourself what is left; well, we'll get to that later. You'll see that there are lots of delicious and healthy foods that will help you to achieve, and maintain, the physique of your dreams.

Valuable tips to lose weight and to remain slender

The following tips will help you achieve the weight of your dreams in a more conscious and positive way:

Eat regularly; that will make you lose weight. You should consume three main meals per day: a balanced breakfast, a lavish lunch, and a light supper. If you just eat these 3 meals, you'll be 100% sure of losing weight optimally. If you want to keep your weight or just lose a little weight, you can include one or two meals in between, to avoid hunger pangs that might occur. Later, in the weekly menus, we will offer both variations.

Eat until you are satisfied; that way, your body won't try to store reserves next time. Try to eat slowly and to chew all your bites well. That way you give your body a chance to tell you when it has received sufficient valuable nutrients.

Drink at least one glass of water before every meal; that will fill the stomach somewhat, and helps achieve an optimal digestion. Drink at least 2.5 liters of water a day. The more water you drink, the better; the high liquid intake promotes the body's detoxification. Avoid drinks that contain sugar; these just increase the blood insulin level.

Try to avoid milk that has a fat content. Milk consists of whey, and whey has the property of increasing the insulin released into the body; combined with the fat it contains, milk is a real fattener. The same applies to other milk products and quark preparations with a high fat contents – it also contains whey.

Coffee and espresso, on the other hand, stimulate the burning of fat, but only if you use stevia instead of the normal sugar, and use low-fat milk. You can drink up to 4 cups of coffee or espresso a day, without harming your body. The coffee's caffeine achieves an increased blood pressure and increases the generation of heat (thermogenesis) in the body, which in turn increases the burning of fat. But bear in mind that for every cup of coffee you should drink a glass of water as compensation.

Stay away from all white flour products, and replace them with whole grain products. This will also increase the fiber content. Use 100% whole grain bread or real whole cereal flakes with fresh fruits for breakfast. Before every lunch or supper, eat a small dish of raw food diet or salad. Avoid white rice and replace it with rice the way it comes from nature; while it is more expensive, it also contains all important nutrients. The same applies to durum wheat noodles; please replace these with whole grain noodles. This might require some getting used to at first, but eventually you'll like the taste of the noodles. You should replace white rice with Basmati rice, brown rice, wild rice or black rice; these still have most nutrients in their shell, as well as fiber.

Please abstain from consuming white (refined) sugar; instead, use stevia. You can also use unrefined cane sugar (just as with the whole grain flour); this can be obtained in specialized bio-shops as well as health food stores. Simple cane sugar, just like white sugar, is not recommended. Here, all minerals and vitamins are removed in the crystallization process, leaving back only unhealthy carbohydrates.

Avoid sweets; the sugar they contain is not recommended, as described above. Better eat fresh fruits or dry fruits. Desserts from the supermarket usually contain white flour and sugar, or butter or margarine, and should therefore also be avoided. If you feel like taking a small piece of chocolate, you can eat one or two pieces now and then; however, the chocolate should have a cocoa content of at least 70%.

Try to move around at least half an hour a day. At first it is always difficult, but you need not get started immediately with power training. Regular training tightens the physique, achieves a good mood, makes your muscles burn more fat cells and benefits your heart and your circulation. The more muscles you have, the more fat will be burned. Every sport activity will re-balance the fat metabolism that got imbalanced. Taking a stroll for half an hour a day will be enough to achieve this. Of course, you can do whatever you find fun; here are some examples: cycling, swimming, aerobics, Pilates, walking, Nordic walking, football, badminton, tennis, stretching, long-distance running, gymnastics, etc. After a while, you'll see that moving really makes you feel well, and that it will also make you lose weight.

Also avoid consuming too much alcohol. A glass of wine at meals is OK, but please don't drink more than that. Also try to abstain from beer; a glass now and then is OK. Alcohol contains 7 kilocalories per gram, and thus twice as much energy as 1 gram of protein. Only fat has more energy at 9 kilocalories. Carbohydrates have 4 kilocalories. Since our body tries to break down alcohol first of all, this will obviously hinder the fat metabolism. Liqueurs and cocktails additionally contain sugar, so it's better to abstain from them completely.

What you should eat at noon, if you don't cook yourself

Many readers won't be able to prepare their own food at noon, and must therefore revert to other options.

If at work you have the option of eating at a cafeteria, bear in mind the following:

Always try to eat a salad dish. A cooked egg combines very well with salad. If vegetables are offered, please take some. Avoid prepared dressings or sauces; these usually contain sauce binders, in other words real fatteners.

With the vegetables you can eat a fish filet, sprinkled with lemon, or you eat filet from chicken, turkey, or veal or beef.

You can also eat tomato with mozzarella, jacket potatoes with herring filet, or jacket potatoes with lean quark.

Always drink only water during the meal; after the meal you can drink an espresso.

As dessert, it is recommended to eat fresh fruits of the season. Abstain from sweet foods such as sweets and creams, which usually contain starch and sugar.

Which additional fat killers you should include in your food, to burn a maximum of fat

Fat killers are foods which greatly increase the metabolism and result in burning fat, since they increase the use of calories. They also preclude the yo-yo effect and reduce the appetite. If you include these fat killers in your food, your fat will dissolve like butter in the sunshine.

Hot spices

Paprika, chili pods (no matter which), cayenne pepper, tabasco, black pepper and other spices to make foods "hot", through the stimulus of the hotness, make the body change to the "thermogenesis" state. In "thermogenesis", also known as heat formation, the metabolism is stimulated; this manifests itself as an increased body temperature. Lots of calories are burned through thermogenesis.

The hotness of paprika fruits is caused by "capsaicin". The capsaicin also has an antibacterial and fungicidal effect. After contact with the hot fruits, be careful not to rub your eyes with your hands; this causes infernal pain.

Cinnamon

Cinnamon regulates insulin and reduces the blood sugar level. The spice also boosts the metabolism and is therefore an excellent fat killer. Less than ½ tea spoon a day is enough to achieve this effect. The best-known and mildest cinnamon is probably the one from Sri Lanka or Ceylon. You can use it to season your cappuccino, but also desserts and main dishes.

Ginger

The ginger root is generally used as a cooking spice; in the Asian region, also as a medicine. The root is strongly antibacterial and has an antiemetic effect, that is, it protects from vomiting. Ginger also promotes circulation, increases the production of bile secretion (this assists digestion) and is considered to be a vegetal aphrodisiac. By increasing the bile secretion, ginger assists digestion and a healthy intestine functioning. Circulation is stimulated through the two ingredients "gingerol" and "shoagol". Similar to the "capsaicin", these stimulate the metabolism through "thermogenesis".

Sauerkraut

Sauerkraut or pickled cabbage is white cabbage conserved through lactic acid fermentation. It is considered to be a national food in Germany. It can be used as garnish or with stews and casseroles. It is rich in fiber and leaves you very satisfied. Sauerkraut is rich in lactic acid, vitamins A, B, C, and K, and minerals, and just like cabbage vegetables in general it is an important native source of vitamin C.

Sauerkraut is very low in calories (ca. 19 kcal per 100 grams), practically fat-free, and contains 3-4% carbohydrates and 1-2% proteins.

Sleep to lose weight?

We already know that half an hour of sports activity per day and a reasonable nutrition are the key to lose weight and to a healthy and vital life.

But how about our sleep? American scientists found, in a study, that sleeping too little reduces the body's basal metabolism, despite the fact that the same amount of calories was consumed. Thus, you should sleep at least 7-8 hours, to have the body influence the metabolism and set it on "saving".

An additional positive effect is achieved by consuming sufficient protein every day, and especially for supper. Protein is a real fat killer. You burn calories after eating foods with legumes, chicken filet, egg white, etc. After eating this, the body needs fat. But when you don't eat fat, the body uses its fat cells. Therefore it is preferable to eat larger amounts of protein in the evening, since the body can then burn its fat cells during the night, at rest.

What you should eat to get slender and maintain your weight effortlessly

Before getting to the recipes, you should know what you can consume for breakfast, to get your body's metabolism up and running.

After getting up, you should drink a glass of lukewarm water; this detoxifies greatly and helps enormously in losing weight. After that you can choose whether you want to eat a 100% whole wheat bread, or rather some other high-value bread (whole grain breads, rye-leaven bread, pumpernickel bread, whole barley bread, soy bread with flax seeds, full grain toast). You can spread this with low-fat fresh cheese or a low-fat granular fresh cheese (max. 0.3% fat). If you prefer it sweet, you can also use sugar-free fruit spread or sugar-free stewed fruit. If you prefer to have it hearty, you can eat turkey or chicken breast (with less than 2% fat contents), or a cooked ham without the fat edge. If you like fish, you might accompany your breakfast with tuna, mackerel, salmon or herring. One thing you can always eat and which helps 100% to lose weight is fresh vegetables such as tomatoes, cucumbers, champignons, carrots, paprika, fennel and salads.

If you prefer to eat muesli for breakfast, you should use full grain corn flakes. You can mix these with some fruit, soy milk, low-fat milk, low-fat quark, or low-fat yoghurt, and if you want to have it sweet, you might add some sugar-free fruit spread or stewed fruit.

A great alternative for breakfast are fruits. Fruits are the perfect ready-made meal, since they are small enough to make a portion, and they are rich in nutrients and sweet.

Most fruits are a great food to take with you, and perfect for those who don't have the time to prepare a sophisticated meal or a snack. However, with fruits there are limitations as well. Only eat bananas occasionally; the same applies to water melon and honeydew melon.

If you want to eat something more sophisticated, make a fruit salad. This can now be purchased in almost any supermarket (make sure that it contains no sugar or aspartame or similar things), or even better (because it will be more fresh) made at home and eaten for breakfast, or as a snack. Two or more fruits, cut into small pieces and mixed, make a fruit salad. Mixing fruits, especially fruits of different colors, supplies us with more nutrients than when we eat a single fruit. Please don't add sugar or a sugar replacement. To sweeten it, just use 1-3 drops of stevia.

You can also use fruit-shakes. Just put several fruits into the mixer and mix them until you get a soft consistency. If the mix is too solid, just add some water. Shakes tend to have more calories than fruits, but they are rich in nutrients and great for anybody who has digestion problems or can't chew hard fruits.

A freshly pressed glass of fruit juice is similar to a shake, but with much less fiber, fruit juice is perfect for anybody with digestion or teeth problems. It's best to press the fruits fresh. However, just like shakes, fruit juices have many calories, so don't drink too many of them.

You can also eat dried fruits with muesli. Dried fruits can be purchased at the store in small and handy packages. While dried fruits don't have the same amount of humidity and nutrients as raw fruits, it is still a great alternative to satisfy our desire for sweet things.

As a drink for breakfast, it is convenient to have a tea or coffee, and a small glass of freshly pressed orange juice. For children, soy milk is recommended, but if you use cocoa powder at all for it, be sure it contains no sugar.

After the breakfast you should wait ca. 2-3 hours before taking your morning snack. If you want to lose weight, forget about the snack, and eat lunch after ca. 4 hours.

The 32 best recipes with vegetables

Vegetables combined with noodles, rice or cheese bring color to your food and usually have valuable power nutrients which keep us satisfied and bring energy into our life.

Try out the following vegetarian meals, and you'll see that you can get satisfied with vegetables as well, while still eating extraordinarily delicious food. Vegetarian vegetable foods will enrapture your palate; you will taste it.

Some recipes include whole grain noodles; these are way healthier than noodles from hard wheat. Unfortunately some people don't like whole wheat noodles; in this case please replace with hard wheat noodles and cook it very firm to bite (al dente).

As mentioned before, you should not use normal rice; it is simply worthless for the body. Please replace it with the specified rice types; these are not only tasty, but they also contain all valuable nutrients which your body needs to lose weight healthily, and not get sick.

Here are some of the abbreviations used:

TBSP = table spoon

TSP = tea spoon

PINCH = pinch (1/16 Teaspoon)

g = grams

Recipes with vegetables and noodles

Wok meal: Broccoli with whole wheat noodles

2 people – time to prepare: 2 minutes – ca. 390 kcal. per person

Ingredients:

500 g broccoli

150 g whole wheat noodles or 150 g noodles al dente

4 bush tomatoes

1 onion

2 cloves of garlic

1 ½ TBSP sesame oil

4 TBSP soy cream

1 TSP Sambal Oelek

1 TBSP freshly grated parmesan

Some sea salt

Some freshly ground pepper

Preparation:

Cook the noodles in abundant lightly salted and boiling water until they are firm to the bite, pour the water off and let it drain. Wash the broccoli, clean it and cut it into small sprouts. Peel the stalks and cut them into small pieces. Peel the onions and the garlic and cut them into small pieces.

Heat the oil in the wok. Fry the broccoli 3-4 minutes while stirring them. Add onions and garlic and continue frying 1-2 more minutes.

Mix with the noodles and season it with some salt, pepper and sambal oelek. Add the soy cream, let it all boil briefly, and then sprinkle it with the freshly grated parmesan. Then distribute on two dishes.

Wash the tomatoes, cut them into four pieces, cut off the stalk and server with the noodles.

Whole grain spaghetti with tomatoes and champignons

2 people – time to prepare: 20 minutes – ca. 410 kcal. per person

Ingredients:

100 g of whole grain spaghetti or 100 g of spaghetti al dente

6 cherry tomatoes

200 g champignons

10 basil leaves

1 clove of garlic

1 TBSP olive oil

Some sea salt

Some freshly ground pepper

1 TBSP freshly grated parmesan

Preparation:

Briefly wash the champignons until they are clean, dry them, remove the stalks and cut them into four pieces. Wash the tomatoes, cut them into four pieces, and remove the stalk.

Peel the garlic and cut it into thin slices. Put a pot with salt water for the spaghetti on the fire, put the pasta into cooking water, and cook it al dente (firm to the bite).

In the meantime, cover the bottom of a pan with olive oil and heat it. Briefly fry the champignons with the garlic in it, then add the tomato quarters. Season it with salt and pepper.

Pour off the water from the pasta, briefly let it drain and put it in the pan. Add finely cut basil leaves and mix everything well.

Prepare dishes with pasta and serve with a bit of freshly grated parmesan.

Whole grain noodles with tofu sauce

4 people – preparation time: 20 minutes – ca. 380 kcal. per person

Ingredients:

250 g whole grain noodles or 250 noodles al dente

400 g tofu

1 onion

1 small clove of garlic

400 ml vegetable broth

2 TBSP sour cream

2 TBSP (flat) of green pesto sauce

1 TBSP olive oil

¼ bunch of parsley

¼ bunch of chives

Sea salt

Freshly ground pepper

Preparation:

Cut the tofu into small pieces and squash it with a fork. Peel the onion and the clove of garlic and cut it into small pieces.

Put the oil into a hot pan and fry the onion and the garlic until they become glassy.

Add the tofu and let it fry for 2 minutes. Pour the broth over it and let the sauce cook covered, at medium heat, for 5 minutes.

Take the pot from the stove and mash it with a blender.

Wash the parsley and the chives, dry it and cut it into small pieces.

Now mix in the sour cream, the pesto and the herbs, and season it with salt and pepper.

In the meantime cook the whole grain noodles in cooking salt water, pour the water off and serve on 4 pasta dishes.

Pour the green tofu sauce on the while wheat noodles and serve directly.

Recipes with vegetables and rice

Tofu curry with basmati rice

4 people – preparation time: 35 min. – ca. 455 kcal. per person

Ingredients:

300 g tofu

1 TBSP sesame oil

2 red paprika

1 bunch of spring onions

800 ml vegetable broth

250 g basmati rice or wild rice

3 TBSP curry paste

1 PINCH hot chili powder

50 g cashew seeds

150 ml coconut milk (unsweetened)

Sea salt

Freshly ground pepper

Preparation:

Wash the paprika pod, dry it, remove the seeds and partitions, and cut it into thin slices.

Wash the spring onions, dry them, and cut them into thin rings.

Heat 2 TBSP of oil in a pot and fry the spring onions with the paprika for ca. 3 minutes in it. Next pour the vegetable broth on it and add the Basmati rice, and let it cook for ca. 20 minutes. After ca. 5 minutes, add the curry paste.

In the meantime, cut the tofu into blocks and heat the remaining oil up in a pan. Roast the tofu together with the cashew seeds.

When the 20 minutes cooking time are over, add the tofu and the cashews to the rice and pour the coconut milk on it. Mix once, and season with salt and pepper; continue adding hot chili powder according to preference, and serve.

Basmati rice with roasted onions and champignons

2 people – preparation time: 35 minutes – ca. 280 kcal. per person

Ingredients:

300 g Basmati rice

600 ml water

300 g fresh champignons

5 onions

2 cloves of garlic

1 TBSP rape oil

400 g natural yoghurt (low-fat yoghurt with 0.3% fat)

1 PINCH paprika powder

Sea salt

Freshly ground pepper

Preparation:

Put the rice with the water into a pot, heat it up, and when it starts to boil, cover it with the lid. Now continue cooking at low heat and with the covered pot, until the water is completely absorbed.

In the meantime clean the champignons and cut them into slices. Peel the onions and the garlic. Cut the onions into rings, press the garlic.

Heat the oil in a pan and roast the onions until they are crispy. Then take the onions out and use the same pan to briefly fry the champignon slices.

Mix the yoghurt with the garlic and season it with salt, pepper and paprika powder.

When the rice is ready, serve on 4 dishes. Put the champignons on top, then the onions, and finally pour the yoghurt on top. Serve directly.

Asian rice and eggplant casserole

2 people – preparation time: 30 minutes – ca. 395 kcal. per person

Ingredients:

150 g whole grain rice

2 small eggplants

½ TSP curcuma

½ TSP curry powder (mild)

½ TSP coriander

1 TBSP lemon juice

100 ml coconut milk

2 TBSP sesame oil

70 g freshly grated parmesan

Some sea salt

Some freshly ground pepper

Preparation:

Put the rice into a pot and add twice as much water, then add the salt. Now let it cook with semi-closed lid until the water is absorbed by the rice.

In the meantime, wash the eggplant, dry it and cut it into finger-thick slices. Sprinkle the lemon juice on it and add some salt. Now let it absorb for 10 minutes.

Next, heat the oil in a pan and slowly fry the eggplant slices. After frying them, take them from the pan and place on a dish.

Pre-heat the oven with circulating air to 200 °C.

When the rice is ready, add the spices and the coconut milk and mix.

Now use a baking-resistant baking dish, add the spiced rice and distribute the eggplant slices on top of it. Sprinkle the cheese on top and let it bake for ca. 10 minutes, then serve.

Risotto, vegetarian version

4 people – preparation time: 35 minutes – ca. 330 kcal. per person

Ingredients:

200 g whole grain wheat

250 g sugar peas

250 g carrots

250 g green beans

500 ml vegetable broth

1 onion

1 TBSP rape oil

1 bunch of parsley

1 PINCH curcuma

Some sea salt

Some freshly ground pepper

Preparation:

Peel the carrots and the onions and cut them into small pieces.

Heat the oil in a pot and fry the onions in it until they get glassy. Add the remaining vegetables and fry for a few minutes. Mix with the rice, pour the broth on it, and season with salt, pepper and curcuma.

Let it cook for ca. 20 minutes on low heat, covered.

Wash the parsley, dry it and cut it into fine pieces, and add to the risotto together with the parmesan. Mix everything well and serve immediately.

Filled eggplants

4 people – preparation time: 30 minutes – ca. 280 kcal. per person

Ingredients:

4 eggplants (ca. 1 kg)

6 tomatoes

200 g Basmati rice or wild rice

500 ml vegetable broth

3 TBSP lemon juice

1 garlic

1 onion

1 bunch of parsley

1 TBSP of rape oil

Some sea salt

Some freshly ground pepper

2 TBSP freshly grated parmesan

Preparation:

Wash the eggplants, cut them in halves with a large kitchen knife, and remove the stalk. With the tip of the peeling knife, free the pulp (the width of a finger from the skin) all around from the skin. Now take the eggplant's pulp out with a spoon, and cut into blocks. Put the pulp in water and leave for ca. 10 minutes, to take out the bitter substances.

Sprinkle the half eggplants with lemon juice, so they don't get brown.

Put a pot with water on the fire and let it boil. Cut into the tomatoes in form a cross, at the end opposite to the stalk. Put them into the water for at most 30 seconds, peel them, take the seeds out and cut the tomatoes into blocks. Peel the onion and the garlic, and cut into small blocks. Wash the parsley, dry it and cut it into fine pieces.

Heat up the oil in a pot and fry the onions and garlic until they get glassy, then add the eggplant pulp and fry it for ca. 3 minutes. Now add the vegetable broth and the rice. If you buy a price that takes longer than 15 minutes to cook, please pre-cook in the broth up to the remaining 15 minutes that come next. Let it cook covered a medium heat, for 15 minutes.

Put the tomatoes briefly into boiling water, peel them, remove the seeds and cut into blocks. Then mix with the chopped parsley.

Pre-heat the oven to 200 degrees.

When the mix of rice and eggplants is cooked, please mix the tomatoes.

Now fill the eggplant halves with the rice mix and put into a casserole form. Put the cheese on top, and cook in the oven for ca. 35-40 minutes with the circulating air procedure at 200 °C. Then put on 4 dishes and serve.

Additional delicious vegetable recipes

Vegetable-Roesti

4 people – preparation time: 30 minutes – ca. 280 kcal. per person

Ingredients:

250 g zucchini

250 g carrots

1 stick of allium

1 small clove of garlic

4 eggs

50 g earthy whole grain oat flakes

1 ½ TBSP rape oil

1 bunch of parsley

1 bunch of chives

Some sea salt

Some freshly ground pepper

Preparation:

Wash the zucchini, dry it, cut it up, remove the seeds and grate it.

Wash the carrots, clean them and grate them.

Wash the stick of allium, clean it, and cut it into thin rings.

Wash the parsley and the chives, dry them and chop them finely.

Open the eggs in a bowl, and mix them with an electrical mixer until they are foamy, then season them with salt and pepper.

Now mix the grated ingredients and the finely chopped ingredients together with the oats in the egg mass.

Heat up the oil in a pan and add 2 TBSP of the rösti mix at a time into the pan, fry both sides until they are golden-brown, and serve immediately.

Fried millet

1 person – preparation time: 45 minutes – ca. 240 kcal. per person

<u>Ingredients:</u>

¼ clove of garlic

¼ onion

A small piece of fresh ginger

1 TBSP rape oil for frying

40 g millet

75 ml instant vegetable broth

40 g carrots

Egg substitute for ¼ egg

Some sea salt

Some chopped parsley

1 TBSP millet flour

Preparation:

Peel the garlic, the onion and the ginger and cut it into small blocks. Heat oil in a pan and fry the onion until it gets glassy, add garlic and ginger. If required, add some salt.

Clean the millet with hot water in a sieve, then put it in the pan and fry it for a few minutes, add the vegetable broth and let the mass cook lightly ca. 15 minutes.

After cooking for 10 minutes, add the finely grated carrot.

The mass must remain on the stove after turning it off for 20 minutes.

Mix the prepared egg replacement mass, the herbs, tomato paste, salt and pepper according to preference. You can also bind the mass with millet meal.

Now, with humid hands, form pieces and fry them with some oil in the pan, on both sides.

Potato and vegetable fritters

1 person – preparation time: 45 minutes – ca. 240 kcal. per person

Ingredients:

200 g potatoes

½ onion

½ stick of allium

1 carrot

Egg substitute for ½ egg (available in health food stores)

1 pinch of marjoram or thyme

Some sea salt

½ teaspoon of potato starch (bio)

Oil for frying

Preparation:

Peel the potatoes and the onions, and grate them finely. Cut the allium lengthwise and cut it into small rings, peel the carrot and grate it finely.

Mix egg substitute according to the manufacturer's instructions. Pour off potato water, if there is any.

Now mix all ingredients with the potato mass, season with marjoram, thyme and salt.

If the mass is too liquid, add some potato starch; this will bind the liquid.

In a coated pan, heat oil and use a teaspoon to put portions of mass into the pan, press them flat and fry them gold-yellow from both sides.

This combines well with a fresh leaf salad.

Vegetable pot with tomatoes

4 people – preparation time: 50 min. – ca. 390 kcal. per person

Ingredients:

4 medium potatoes

4 large carrots

2 small fennel tubers

2 small zucchini

1 branch of rosemary

1 branch of thyme

3 cloves of garlic

2 onions

5 TBSP olive oil

Some sea salt

Some black pepper

¼ l vegetable broth

4 beef tomatoes

2 small, round goat cheeses (20 g each)

1 bunch of dill

Preparation:

Peel the potatoes and the carrots, clean the fennel and the zucchini, cut all in blocks of appropriate size. Strip rosemary and onions and chop them finely.

Fry all vegetables separately, in each case with 1 teaspoon of oil, and season with some rosemary, thyme, garlic, salt and pepper. Mix everything in the pan and add vegetable broth. Let it cook open for ca. 10 minutes, until the liquid evaporates.

In the meantime, peel tomatoes, take out their seeds, and cut them into large pieces. Add salt and pepper. Crumble the goat cheese and mix it with the tomatoes. Disperse over the vegetables, take pan from stove, and leave it covered for ca. 5 minutes.

Chop the dill and disperse it over the food.

Tomatoes filled with quark

1 person – preparation time: 20 minutes – ca. 280 kcal. per person

Ingredients:

3 large tomatoes

3 black olives

1 onion

2 cloves of garlic

Some basil

A few drops wine vinegar

1 teaspoon of olive oil

125 g low-fat quark

Some sea salt

Some freshly ground pepper

Preparation:

Wash the tomatoes, cut a sort of lid out and scoop them out. Cut the scooped-out tomato pulp and the olives into small pieces, also cut the chives, basil, onion and garlic and add it.

Add the wine vinegar and the olive oil, and mix with the low-fat quark, spice it with iodized salt or sea salt as well as pepper. With this mix of quark and vegetables you fill out the hollowed tomatoes. Finally, put the lid you cut off previously back on.

Jacket potatoes with herb quark

4 people – preparation time: 30 minutes – ca. 400 kcal. per person

Ingredients:

1000 g small potatoes

500 g low-fat quark

100 ml low-fat milk

1 bunch of chives

1 bunch of parsley

1 PINCH cayenne pepper

Some sea salt

Some freshly ground pepper

Preparation:

Thoroughly wash the potatoes, cook them in salt water, let them cook until they are well cooked in 20-25 minutes and pour the water off. Let the potatoes' vapors escape in an open pot, while shaking it frequently. Now mix the quark with the milk.

Wash the chives and the parsley, dab them dry, chop them finely and mix them with the quark. Season with salt, pepper and cayenne pepper, and beat until it is fluffy.

Make a lengthwise cut in the potatoes, press them open and add 1 teaspoon of the quark with herbs, then serve. You can also peel the potatoes and serve with the quark.

Jacket potatoes and carrots in the pan

4 people – preparation time: 30 minutes – ca. 390 kcal. per person

Ingredients:

700 g small potatoes

300 g carrots

1 clove of garlic

3 eggs

50 ml low-fat milk

2 TBSP rape oil

½ bunch of parsley

½ bunch of chives

1 TBSP rosemary

1 TSP liquid honey

200 ml vegetable broth

2 TBSP rape oil

100 g Harz cheese

Some sea salt

Some freshly ground pepper

Preparation:

Thoroughly clean the potatoes, wash them, cook them in salt water, leave them 20-25 minutes until they are cooked, and pour off the water. Let the potatoes' vapors escape in an open pot, while shaking it frequently.

In the meantime, brush the carrots thoroughly and wash them, peel them thin, cut off and remove both ends, then cut diagonally into thin slices. Peel the garlic cloves and press them.

Heat up 1 TBSP of oil in a pan and swivel the carrot slices together with the garlic in it for about 3 minutes.

Add the rosemary and the honey to the carrots and mix everything well.

Quickly pour some vegetable broth on it and let it cook ca. 5-7 minutes more until it is firm to the bite; if necessary, add some more liquid. Then take the carrots out of the pan and take the remaining liquid out of the pan.

Now cut the jacket potatoes into slices; if the potatoes break apart while doing this, that's no problem.

Cut the Harz cheese up into small pieces.

Wash the parsley and chives, dry them, and chop them finely.

Open the eggs and put them in a container with the milk, season with some salt and pepper and beat with a hand whisk until it is foamy.

In the pan, heat 1 TBSP of oil, add the carrots and the potatoes and pour the egg mass over it. Now mix, and wait until the eggs start to stagnate. Then sprinkle the herbs (except for a small remainder) and the cheese over it and mix briefly, to distribute the cheese well. Continue stagnating at low heat until the egg mass is solid, then serve directly and sprinkle the remaining herbs over it.

I hope that you like the book so far. If you have ideas or comments, you can always find me at:

I would be happy to get a well-written review at Amazon or any other book vendor.

Now, let's continue with the delicious recipes to lose weight.

Lasagna with vegetables and cheese

2 people – preparation time: 25 minutes – ca. 350 kcal. per person

Ingredients:

100 g Harz cheese

200 g cottage cheese (low-fat level)

4 tomatoes

200 g fresh champignons

1 onion

1 egg

2 slices of cooking ham without fat border

Preparation:

Pre-heat the oven to 200 °C, with circulating air.

Peel the onion and cut it into blocks. Cut the ham into thin strips and cut the Harz cheese into small blocks.

Now put all the ingredients together with the opened egg into a bowl and mix vigorously until everything is mixed.

Put the mix into an oven mold and bake completely for ca. 20 minutes. Take it out of the oven, put it on 2 dishes and serve directly.

Toscana Spinach

2 people – preparation time: 20 minutes – ca. 280 kcal. per person

Ingredients:

3 TBSP unsulfured apricots

400 g fresh leaf spinach

1 small onion

1 TBSP rape oil

25 g pine nuts

Some sea salt

Some freshly grated nutmeg

3 TBSP low-fat yoghurt

Preparation:

Soak the apricots in lukewarm water. Carefully pick the spinach, clean it, wash it and chop it coarsely. Peel the onion and cut it up very finely.

Melt the butter in a pot and fry the onion blocks in it until they get glassy. Add the spinach and let it collapse.

In the meantime, roast the pine nuts in a pan without adding fat, until they have a golden-brown color. Let the raisins drain and add them together with the pine nuts to the spinach. Season with salt and nutmeg. Finally add some low-fat yoghurt to the spinach. Mix everything well, and let it steam 5 more minutes at medium heat.

Fried asparagus with parmesan

1 person – preparation time: 25 minutes – ca. 330 kcal. per person

Ingredients:

250 g asparagus

½ bunch of parsley

2 dried tomatoes

1 TBSP sesame oil

Some sea salt

Some fresh pepper

10 g grated parmesan cheese

Preparation:

Peel the asparagus and briefly fry it in a pan with the sesame oil, season with iodized salt or sea salt and pepper, then add ca. 100 ml water and let it cook with the lid on, for 15-20 minutes.

Chop the chives and the dried tomatoes finely, take the asparagus out, let the broth cook a while and then add the tomatoes and the chives, let it cook on low heat for a few minutes.

Pour the herb broth over the asparagus and slice the parmesan cheese over it.

As a side dish, you can use a small beef steak (without fat) and a whole grain toast.

Filled zucchini

4 people – preparation time: 30 minutes – ca. 290 kcal. per person

<u>Ingredients:</u>

4 large or 8 small zucchini

1 paprika pod (red or yellow)

4 TSP macadamia oil

½ bunch of parsley

12 black olives without their seeds

8 macadamia nuts

2 TSP of freshly grated parmesan

Some sea salt

Some freshly ground pepper

Preparation:

Start by pre-heating the oven to 180 °C. Cut the zucchini lengthwise into halves and hollow them out with a small spoon; keep the pulp. Next blanch the zucchini halves for a few minutes. To blanch vegetables, they are briefly placed in hot water, then poured over with cold water.

Wash the paprika pod, dry it, removes seeds and partitions and cut it into small blocks, and steam it together with the zucchini pulp in a small pot, with olive oil.

Then chop the olives and the macadamia into small pieces.

Wash the parsley, dry it and chop it into small pieces.

Mix the chopped olives and macadamia with the cheese and season with parsley as well as salt and pepper.

Now mix the previously cooked zucchini with the vegetable mix and finish baking it in a bake-resistant non-sticking form for 15 minutes, then serve directly.

Breaded cauliflower with potatoes

4 people – preparation time: 35 minutes – ca. 435 kcal. per person

Ingredients:

800 g of small potatoes

1 large cauliflower

1 egg

1 TSP breadcrumbs

1 piece of butter

1 SS olive oil

1 TSP cumin

1 bunch of parsley

Some sea salt

Some freshly ground pepper

Preparation:

Wash the parsley, dry it and chop it. Wash the potatoes and cook them until they are well cooked in a top with salt and cumin. The potatoes are cooked when, if you pierce them with a sharp knife, they slip back off the knife.

In the meantime, clean the cauliflower, cut it up into relatively small sprouts and cook it in salt water until it is firm to the bite. When they cool down, roll the cauliflower sprouts first in egg then in bread crumbs, and fry them in butter until they have a nice gold-brown color.

Pour off the water from the cooked potatoes and briefly cool them down with cold water; that way, they are easier to peel. Fry the peeled potatoes whole in a pan with the olive oil, at medium heat. When they start getting light-brown, add the chopped parsley and let them fry for a while longer. Season with salt and pepper and serve together with the cauliflower.

White bean soufflé

2 people – preparation time: 110 minutes – pre-preparation time 1 night – ca. 440 kcal. per person

Ingredients:

100 g white beans

4 tomatoes

150 ml low-fat milk

4 eggs

1 onion

1 TBSP thyme

1 TBSP parsley

1 TSP rosemary

Some sea salt

Some freshly ground pepper

Preparation:

First, the beans should be soaked, preferably overnight, and then cooked with the soaking water and some salt for 90 minutes. Then mash the beans with a fork.

Peel the onion and cut it into fine blocks, and mix it with the milk and the mashed beans.

Wash the tomatoes, cut them into quarters, remove the stalk, then cut them into small pieces. Make the bean mass cook, then add the tomatoes and the herbs. Season with salt and pepper.

Pre-heat the oven with circulating air to 180 °C.

Open the 4 eggs and separate the egg white and the yolk. Beat the egg white until it is stiff, then mix it with the bean mass.

Put the bean mass into a big baking form and leave the soufflé in the oven for 1 hour at 180 °C. Then take it out, and serve it.

Vegetable skewer

2 people – preparation time: 20 minutes; marinating time: ca. 120 minutes – ca. 350 kcal. per person

Ingredients:

1 zucchini

1 small eggplant

1 small red paprika pod

200 g champignons

1 onion

100 g apricots

2 branches of oregano

50 ml macadamia oil (sunflower oil)

Some Himalaya salt or sea salt

Some ground black pepper

Preparation:

Wash the zucchini and the eggplant, clean it, and cut it into slices, one finger thick. Cut the eggplant slices in two.

Cut the paprika hull in two, clean it, wash it and cut it into large pieces. Wash the champignons or rub them with a cloth. Peel the onion, cut it into four parts, and separate it into layers. Cut the apricots in halves (removing the stones), wash them hot and dry them well.

Put all the ingredients in a row on a metal or wooden spike. Put the spikes close together in a flat, rectangular bowl.

Wash the oregano, dry it and take the leaves from the stems. Whisk the herb leaves with the oil, season this with salt and pepper and sprinkle it on the vegetable sprouts. Leave the sprouts covered and let them marinate ca. 2 hours.

To serve, pre-heat a grill. Lay the spikes on the grill grid and let them get brown all around below or above the hot grill. Now and then, sprinkle them with the marinating sauce.

Green beans à la Ceylon

4 people – preparation time: 35 minutes – ca. 335 kcal. per person

Ingredients:

800 g fresh green beans

400 g tomatoes

5 cloves of garlic

100 ml mineral water (without carbonic acid)

300 ml vegetable broth

1 walnut-sized ginger

1 red chili pod

4 TBSP sesame oil

2 TSP ground cumin

2 TSP coriander

2 TSP curcuma

2 TBSP lemon juice (from fresh lemons)

Some sea salt

Some freshly ground pepper

Preparation:

Briefly put the tomatoes in hot water, peel them, take out the seeds and cut into blocks.

Cut the chili pod into halves, take out the seeds and partition walls, wash it, dry it and cut it into very small pieces. Please wash your hands thoroughly after that.

Wash the green beans, dry them, take out their threads and cut off the ends. Then cut them into pieces of about 1 cm each.

Peel the ginger and the garlic and put them into a high container with ca. 100 ml water, and use the blender to convert them into a paste.

Slightly heat the oil in a pan and fry the cumin with the chili pieces until the chili pieces get slightly darker. Now add the paste and mix. After a minute, add the tomato pieces, and continue mixing for a minute. Now add the coriander and the curcuma, and pour the vegetable broth on the beans.

Add the lemon juice, abundant pepper and some salt.

Take the lid off, and cook on low heat until the liquid disappears. Frequently stir the beans, to avoid them from sticking to the base. In between, season with salt and pepper. As soon as the liquid disappears, you should serve it.

Allium with saffron

4 people – preparation time: 45 minutes – ca. 320 kcal. per person

Ingredients:

14 allium sticks

5 tomatoes

10 thyme twigs

1 bunch of parsley

4 cloves of garlic

1 onion

3 TBSP olive oil

100 ml dry white wine

1 PINCH ground saffron

Some sea salt

Some ground black pepper

Preparation:

Clean the allium; to do this, cut off the white root beginning and the upper ¼ of the green part. Thoroughly wash the sticks and cut them into pieces of ca. 5 cm each.

Incise the tomatoes in a cross, briefly put them into boiling water, rinse with cold water, and peel them. Cut them into four pieces, take out the seeds and cut them into large pieces.

Wash the thyme and the parsley and shake them dry. Peel the garlic and, together with the parsley, chop them finely.

Heat up the olive oil in a large pot and fry the onions at medium heat until they get brown. Then add the allium, the tomatoes, and the parsley-garlic mix, and also let it get slightly brown.

Now add the white wine, the saffron and some salt and pepper. Pull off the thyme leaves over the pot and stir. Let everything cook on low heat for ca. 20 minutes. The allium should still have some bite. Season the allium, serve it warm or cold.

Leaf spinach and turnip casserole

<ins>Ingredients:</ins>

250 g leaf spinach

1 turnip head

2 tomatoes

50 g ground Gouda cheese

150 g soy crème fraiche or normal crème fraiche

Some freshly ground nutmeg

1 onion

2 TBSP rape oil

2 TBSP chopped parsley

Some sea salt

Some freshly ground pepper

Preparation:

Briefly place the tomatoes into hot water, peel them, take the seeds out and cut them into pieces. Peel the onion and cut it into fine pieces.

Peel the turnip and cut it into blocks, then cook it for 3 minutes in boiling salt water. Then cook the spinach in the turnip water and let it collapse, and rinse it with cold water.

Let the turnip and spinach drain and stack it on an oven-resistant casserole form.

Pre-heat the oven with circulating air at 200 °C.

Stir the cheese with the soy crème fraiche and season it with salt, pepper and nutmeg, then sprinkle it over the vegetables.

Put the casserole into the oven and bake it for ca. 15-20 minutes. In the meantime, heat up oil in a pan and fry the onion until it gets glassy. Then add the tomatoes and let it cook for ca. 5 minutes at low heat. Season it with salt and pepper, sprinkle the parsley on it and mix it.

When the casserole is golden-brown, take it out of the oven, pour the tomato sauce over it and serve.

Tomato and sheep cheese casserole

2 people – preparation time: 35 minutes – ca. 310 kcal. per person

Ingredients:

4 tomatoes

150 g sheep cheese (mild)

½ orange

1 clove of garlic

8 basil leaves

½ bunch of parsley

4 thyme twigs

½ TSP rosemary

2 TBSP olive oil

Some sea salt

Some freshly ground pepper

Preparation:

Wash the tomatoes, dry them and cut them into slices; while doing this, remove the stalk.

Press out the half oranges and save the juice.

Cut the sheep cheese into thin slices.

Wash the parsley and the thyme, dry it and chop it finely.

Peel the garlic and press it. Now mix the garlic with the herbs, the olive oil and the orange juice and stir it well, then season with salt and pepper.

Pre-heat the oven with circulating air at 180 °C.

In an oven-resistant casserole form, put alternating layers of tomato and cheese slices on top of each other, and pour some orange and oil dressing on each layer.

Bake the casserole 15-20 minutes in the oven; please don't let the cheese get dark. Then get it out and decorate it with the washed and dried basil leaves, and serve.

Brussels sprouts

4 people – preparation time: 35 minutes – ca. 250 kcal. per person

Ingredients:

500 g Brussels sprouts

2 onions

2 TBSP rape oil

1 PINCH grated nutmeg

40 g almond leaves

Some sea salt

Some freshly ground pepper

Preparation:

Briefly wash the Brussels sprouts and with a small, pointy knife remove 2-3 outer leaves and the stems from each. Incise the ends in a cross, to let the sprouts cook quicker and more uniformly. In a pot, boil a small amount of slightly salted water. Add the Brussels sprouts and let them cook in a covered pot for ca. 20 minutes, until they are firm to bite. Peel the onions and cut them into very fine pieces.

Melt the oil in a small pan and fry the onions in it. Add the almonds and fry them until the color changes to brown. Then take the pan from the stove. Put the Brussels sprouts into a sieve and let them drain. Put them back into the pot. Add the almonds and onions, and mix with the oil. Then season the Brussels sprouts with salt, pepper, grated nutmeg and the lemon juice. Serve directly.

This combines very well with the fried jacket potatoes from the recipe of the breaded cauliflower.

Vegetarian hand cheese

4 people – preparation time: 25 minutes – ca. 210 kcal. per person

Ingredients:

1 eggplant

1 zucchini

6 bush tomatoes

2 onions

2 cloves of garlic

250 g hand cheese with cumin

10 green olives (without stones)

1 stem of thyme

½ bunch of parsley

12 basil leaves

2 TBSP balsamic vinegar

1 TBSP rape oil

Some sea salt

Some freshly ground pepper

Preparation:

Clean the zucchini and the eggplant and cut them into blocks.

Peel the onions and the garlic; cut the onions into thin slices and press the garlic. Wash the tomatoes, dry them and cut them into slices, removing the stalk.

Wash the herbs, dry them and cut them finely. Cut the olives into slices.

Heat the oil in a pot, and fry the onions and garlic for about a minute. Now sprinkle the vegetable pieces and fry for an additional 5 minutes. Then sprinkle the olives and the herbs over the tomatoes and stir. Now add the vinegar and season with salt and pepper.

Cut the cheese into thin slices, distribute on 4 dishes and distribute the vegetables over it.

Potato dumplings

4 people – preparation time: 50 minutes – ca. 100 kcal. per person

Ingredients:

500 grams of cooked jacket potatoes

1 egg

1 onion

5 TBSP breadcrumbs

5 TBSP of potato flour

Some nutmeg

1 TBSP chopped parsley

Some butter

Some sea salt

Preparation:

Peel the onions and chop them very finely, or press them. Scrub the jacket potatoes and wash them, then cook them in salt water until they are cooked. Potatoes are cooked when, if you stick a pointy knife into them, they slip back off.

Peel the potatoes and mash them, mix with the flour, the egg and the breadcrumbs. Season with parsley, nutmeg and salt. Shape the mass into balls, briefly parboil them and then leave them cooking slowly. In total, they should boil ca. 15-20 minutes. Then take them out of the water and serve directly.

Asian vegetable wok

2 people – preparation time: 20 minutes – ca. 220 kcal. per person

Ingredients:

2 yellow paprika

3 carrots

3 tomatoes

3 spring onions

3 cloves of garlic

300 g broccoli

1 ginger, the size of a hazelnut

½ red chili pod

3 TBSP soy sauce

1 TBSP lemon juice

2 TBSP sesame oil

1 TSP liquid honey

1 PINCH cinnamon

Some sea salt

Some freshly ground white pepper

Preparation:

Wash the broccoli, remove the stalk and separate it into small sprouts. Clean the carrots and cut them into thin slices. Cook the carrots and the broccoli together in a pot with salt water for ca. 6 minutes, then pour the water off.

In the meantime, wash the tomatoes, dry them, divide them into eight pieces each, removing the stalks. Wash the paprika, dry it, cut it open, remove the inside and cut it into slices. Clean the spring onions, wash them, dry them and cut them into thin slices. Peel the ginger and the cloves of garlic and chop them finely. Then thoroughly wash your hands.

Heat the oil very hot in the wok or in a high pan, and briefly fry the ginger, the garlic and the chili. Now add the vegetables and add the soy sauce. While continuously stirring, continue frying ca. 3-5 minutes (depending on your preferences). Finally add the honey and season with salt and pepper, then serve directly.

Various vegetable sauces

Coconut sauce

2 people – preparation time: ca. 10 minutes – ca. 150 kcal. per person

Ingredients:

¼ onion

¼ clove of garlic

Margarine for frying

100 ml coconut drink

1 small piece of ginger

1 pinch of curcuma

1 small piece of cinnamon stick

Some sea salt

Some freshly ground pepper

Preparation:

Peel the onion and the garlic and cut it into small blocks, then, in a pan with margarine, fry the onion and the garlic until it is glassy, add the coconut milk, let it cook briefly, add the finely grated ginger, curcuma, and the piece of cinnamon stick, season with salt and pepper.

Before serving, you must remove the cinnamon stick. This sauce combines well with all sorts of vegetables, as well as fowl and fish.

Broccoli sauce

4 people – preparation time: ca. 20 minutes – ca. 160 kcal. per person

Ingredients:

¼ onion

125 g broccoli

1 tablespoon of oil

1 knife tip of granulated vegetable broth

100 ml oats drink plus calcium

½ tablespoon of oats flakes

Some sea salt

Some freshly ground pepper

Preparation:

Peel the onion and cut it into small blocks, wash the broccoli and separate it into small sprouts. Heat up the oil in a pot, and fry the onions until they get glassy, add the broccoli and pour a quarter cup of water on top, add the granulated vegetable broth. Let the broccoli cook lightly, covered, for ca. 5 minutes.

Then add the oats drink and let it cook once more for ca. 10 minutes, then crush everything finely with a blender. Season with pepper and salt. If the sauce is too thin, it can be thickened with instant oat flakes.

The sauce is great for noodle meals, but it also tastes well with rice or a salad.

Pea sauce

2 people – preparation time: ca. 15 minutes – ca. 160 kcal. per person

Ingredients:

¼ onion

1 tablespoon of oil

25 ml instant vegetable broth

25 ml rice drink

75 g frozen peas

Some sea salt

Some freshly ground white pepper

¼ apricot

Preparation:

Peel the onion and cut it into small pieces, fry the onion in a pot with oil until it gets glassy, add the vegetable broth, the rice drink and the peas and let it all cook ca. 10 minutes at low heat.

Mash the mass into a fine sauce and season it with salt and pepper.

Wash the apricot, remove the stones and cut the apricot into small pieces. Before serving, it can be mixed with the sauce, or it can be sprinkled on top to enhance the color. This sauce is great for potato meals, but it also combines well with rice or noodle meals.

www.ingramcontent.com/pod-product-compliance
Lightning Source LLC
Chambersburg PA
CBHW070806290526
45795CB00002B/646